Power-Full Weight Loss

M.Grace

BALBOA.
PRESS

A DIVISION OF HAY HOUSE

Balboa Press books may be ordered through booksellers or by contacting:

Balboa Press
A Division of Hay House
1663 Liberty Drive
Bloomington, IN 47403
www.balboapress.com
1-(877) 407-4847

ISBN: 978-1-4525-4920-0 (sc)
ISBN: 978-1-4525-4921-7 (hc)
ISBN: 978-1-4525-4919-4 (e)

Library of Congress Control Number: 2012905612

Because of the dynamic nature of the Internet, any web addresses or links contained in this book may have changed since publication and may no longer be valid. The views expressed in this work are solely those of the author and do not necessarily reflect the views of the publisher, and the publisher hereby disclaims any responsibility for them.

The author of this book does not dispense medical advice or prescribe the use of any technique as a form of treatment for physical, emotional, or medical problems without the advice of a physician, either directly or indirectly. The intent of the author is only to offer information of a general nature to help you in your quest for emotional and spiritual well-being. In the event you use any of the information in this book for yourself, which is your constitutional right, the author and the publisher assume no responsibility for your actions.

Any people depicted in stock imagery provided by Thinkstock are models, and such images are being used for illustrative purposes only.
Certain stock imagery © Thinkstock.

Printed in the United States of America

Balboa Press rev. date: 6/4/2012

Contents

Foreword

This book has been written to offer motivation and support to those who are struggling to lose unwanted weight and to adopt a healthier lifestyle. It allows the reader to understand that I too have experienced the struggle of being obese and I can therefore offer realistic guidance as to how your weight loss can be achieved and maintained, your health restored and your confidence boosted.

The prospect of change can seem scary, but every step you take will become easier than the last!

You obviously want to change; otherwise you wouldn't be reading this book. Change the word 'want' to 'will' and you will find that your dreams *will* become a reality!

Good luck

Margaret Grace
April 2012

Introduction

"Who am I?" This is a question most people ask at some point in their life. If you are reflective, like me, then you've probably asked this question several times. I describe myself as being reflective because I feel that this helps me to describe the type of person I am. I am a person who thinks about things; I analyze situations, body language and my own emotions and then I try to make sense of why things are the way they are.

When I was younger, my mum used to say that I thought too much. I must say that it's only now, as an adult, that I can appreciate why my mum made that comment. What my mum was noticing was not that I thought too much, but rather that my thoughts were not helpful. I over-analyzed things and had unhelpful thoughts that eventually became destructive to my emotional, spiritual and mental well-being. Other people at that time may have described me as being too sensitive, over-emotional, or lacking in confidence. Perhaps these are words that you would use to describe yourself.

Despite the fact that such thoughts did welcome utter chaos into my life, I do not resent the fact that I am reflective, nor do I regret my past experiences. Instead, I feel blessed because I have allowed my thinking to become more positive and more mature. Whilst I still have a deep awareness of situations and the actions and intentions of other people, I have grown up and become more objective in the way that I handle my thoughts.

Instead of being over-sensitive and assuming that an event has happened because I am not good enough, I am not likeable, I'm too fat, I've made a mistake, I'm too ugly, et cetera, I can now empathize with other people and understand that the event happened because of some other factor which is not my fault! I also appreciate now that I am just as worthy as other people, I am as special as everyone else and my opinions do count. This awareness has also allowed me to recognise that other people are also vulnerable and those people who appear to be confident are often not as confident as they project. I am in no way suggesting that all people are secretly weak individuals lacking in confidence, but I am suggesting that there is a vulnerability that exists in all of us. Recognising this has allowed me to understand that I am 'normal' and that this vulnerability can be the cause of the way in which people act. I believe that provided we follow our instincts and act accordingly, things in life do happen for a reason. It sounds clichéd, but I believe it to be true.

What I have also grown to learn is that whilst some of the difficulties we face in life may be the result of other people's mistakes, we actually have more control in such situations than we think. This is because, as human beings, we are able to choose the way we feel and respond to different situations. If we are feeling sad, then that is because we *choose* to feel sad and if we feel fat and unattractive, that is because we *choose* to feel fat and unattractive. Once we really understand this, we are able to regain peace, harmony and control in our lives. We can be who we are really meant to be and *choose* to feel positive because we know it feels right. To feel positive, we know that it feels right to think positive thoughts: 'I feel happy' or 'I feel slim and attractive.'

The trouble is that so many of us fail to recognise what our instincts are telling us and we make decisions that are not in harmony with our individual beings. People make mistakes and life can become really tough. It's during these tough times that we reflect and realise we haven't been listening to or loving ourselves the way we should. We resolve to change and as we do, we develop a greater awareness of ourselves, our needs and our ability to succeed.

If you feel a bit lost, as if you're hiding behind a layer of fat and people don't know the real you, don't despair. I've been where you are. I understand how lonely and isolating being overweight can be. I can recall

- struggling to bend down to tie my shoelaces;
- feeling sadness, embarrassment, anger and hatred whenever I looked at my reflection;
- avoiding social situations because I had nothing to wear and feared being the only fat person at a function;
- getting out of breath when I walked—never mind going up a flight of stairs; and
- feeling embarrassed when I struggled to fit my bottom between the arm rests of a seat on a train or aeroplane.

I *hated* feeling all of these things. It was awful, it wasn't right, it wasn't healthy and it wasn't me. I vowed to change . . . and I did. You can change, too.

Things may seem really awful just now, but if you follow the advice in this book and the help that a health professional gives you, you will be able to get rid of the excess weight and become both physically and mentally stronger. Now doesn't that sound great?

Part I of this book shares my knowledge and advice to achieving weight loss. It is essential that you read this section carefully and consider the information given. Whilst you probably will not do things exactly the same way, you should aim to apply the underlying principals and tactics I have used to suit your own lifestyle. (This will become clear as you progress through each section).

I have divided Part I of the book into three sections. Each section focuses on a different topic that is in some way relevant to weight loss and healthy living. You can dip in and out of each section and write notes in the margin or at the end of the section.

Part II helps you to devise a weight loss plan that is unique and tailored to your needs. We are all different so it is important that you have a plan that compliments *your* lifestyle and values.

Part III has a section called 'Other Information, Advice & Support', which lists organizations and websites that you may find to be beneficial.

Just remember—this is *your* life. Do this for you—no one else!

PART I

Getting Started

In order to make any significant change in your life, you need to take time to figure out what your motives are for changing. You also need to ask yourself if you really *want* to change. If you read this section, answer the questions and find that for whatever reason you are not ready to change, don't worry. Just as a smoker may contemplate giving up smoking for months or years before actually doing so—perhaps having several failed attempts, a person who is trying to lose weight may think about it for a long time and also have several failed attempts before achieving success.

Both the person giving up smoking and the person wanting to lose weight will eventually achieve the success that she desires, provided that she does it for herself *and* she believes that she can succeed. (Don't worry if you do doubt yourself; I'll tell you how to believe in yourself later)!

First ensure that you have some privacy, then get yourself a sheet of paper, a pen, and a ruler. Draw a table on the paper with the following column titles:

- Reasons for Losing Weight
- Reasons for Not Losing Weight

Complete your table as honestly as you can. This is a personal exercise—no one is going to see this sheet, so just go for it!

Below, is an example of a table similar to the one I completed at the start of my journey.

Reasons for Losing Weight	Reasons for Not Losing Weight
• Feel happier • Feel healthier—back won't be sore, normal blood pressure, good skin/hair, less tired • Look healthier • Look sexier • Feel sexier • More confidence and motivation to go out and meet people • Wear whatever I want • Won't be restricted to a few clothes shops that cater for plus sizes • Do up my shoelaces, put on my socks with ease • Fasten seat belts • Fit in seats • Won't feel embarrassed • Won't have to try to disguise the fact that I'm out of breath after climbing stairs etc whilst with company	• Can eat what I want • Can eat when I want • Don't have to think about how much fat/ sugar I'm eating • Don't have to think about taking more exercise • Don't have to be bothered with the hassle of losing weight

If you're like me, you'll find that your 'reasons for' section could go on and on and that the 'reasons for not' section has 'reasons' that really hold no value or substance. You'll probably find that one of your first reasons for losing weight is to feel happier. This reason to me is the most significant and important reason for wanting to lose weight.

Because your physical and mental health are influenced by each other, it is obvious that if your physical health is suffering, your mental health will suffer too. That is, you'll very likely suffer from depression, feel sad, have an arrogant attitude, despise yourself and more. Once you reach your ideal weight for optimum health, you will feel happier, too.

Next, get a new sheet of paper and write down your reasons why you think that you've failed to lose weight in the past. Leave a couple of lines between each section. Again, these responses should be personal and honest. Some reasons that I wrote down are detailed below.

- *Fear*—I was afraid of changing what had become a 'normal' way of life for me and I was afraid of what I would become. I was afraid that I wouldn't achieve my goals and would end up feeling like a failure. I was also afraid that things I did not expect to change (e.g., friendships, my attitudes towards different issues in life) would change.

- *Lack of Motivation*—Since I failed to notice instant results and had strong cravings for sugary foods following a couple of days of 'strict dieting', I would lose motivation and return to my unhealthy and familiar habits.

- *Social Distractions*—Events like birthdays and meals out with friends meant that just as I was trying really hard to adopt healthier habits, the temptation to indulge in foods that I had not intended to eat on a particular day proved too great whenever any of these social occasions arose.

- *Boredom and Cravings*—Too often I would get fed up with eating the same restrictive diet day after day. Such boredom would exacerbate cravings for high-calorific foods such as chocolate and I would end up bingeing on large quantities of these foods.

Once you have completed your list, carefully examine each statement and consider carefully how these problems could be overcome. For example, since I listed fear as one of the obstacles that previously interfered with my progress, I would have to consider how this feeling could be changed into a positive emotion so that it could aid and not hinder my progress. I asked myself to confirm exactly what I was afraid of. One of the things I feared was that my friendships would change as I achieved my goal. In an attempt to deal with this, I acknowledged that I had no proof to suggest that my friendships would change. However if they did change, I had to also acknowledge that such relationships could, in fact, intensify and strengthen. (If this was to happen, then I would be very fortunate to achieve not only a healthier version of myself but a firmer friendship, too!) If my friendships changed in a negative way, then I would have to question whether such friends were really the type of friends that I needed in my life and who truly had my best interests at heart. I knew that due to a friend's jealousy or my increasing confidence, this situation could be a reality, but even if it were to happen, it would very likely happen over a period of time, thus allowing me to mentally accept that a friendship was coming to an end.

Understandably what it was that I feared and whether or not such fears were justified, allowed me to deal with the problem in a logical way. I was also then able to focus on changing the feeling of fear into a feeling of excitement. It wasn't easy to start with, but after a bit of perseverance, I got there!

Following this process, you must reflect on each of your other obstacles that have hindered your progress previously. Carefully consider their significance and how they could be overcome. Whilst I would encourage you to not become bogged down by this process, you must not skip it or rush it, either. I'm sure that most overweight people would agree that weight loss cannot simply be achieved by eating less. It is more complex, requiring an individual to reflect, question, discover and adapt. What you think and how you deal with your thoughts has a *huge* significance on your ability to achieve your goals. You must strive to think positive thoughts about yourself and believe in your ability to achieve your goals. You must learn to acknowledge any negative feelings or emotions, questioning their significance and if they are prompting you to change something. Then you must let go of the negative feelings and experience positive thoughts and feelings instead. If you don't believe in yourself and continue to feel negative, you will lack the motivation and determination to succeed.

If you're struggling to believe in yourself, just pretend that you do. Practise saying positive affirmations to yourself (e.g., 'I am a healthy size. I nourish my body with healthy foods. I deserve to be a healthy weight'). Say these affirmations out loud and in front of a mirror. Close your eyes and visualise yourself at your ideal weight. Focus really hard on feeling what it's like being this weight. Do your affirmations and visualisations every day. Both exercises are very powerful and I will speak more about them later. Eventually these positive affirmations can be practised effortlessly and you will find that you do believe in yourself and that your goals will become a reality!

Believe in yourself. You *can* achieve your goal—other people have, so why can't you? You're no different, I promise. Go for it—at least give it a try!

After completing your 'reasons for' table and your list of obstacles, you must get a diary and keep these notes in your diary. This diary is your conscience, memory and mentor throughout your regime. You *must*, on a daily basis, write down exactly what you have eaten and drank. You must also write down any exercise that you have done. On a weekly basis (no more frequently), write down your weight (or your measurements; measurements are discussed in greater detail in the next section).

If you're following a calorie—or fat-controlled diet, you may wish to write down these values next to your daily food consumption with a total written at the end of each day. Or if you have chosen to follow a reputable diet regime such as Weight Watchers, you may wish to record points instead of calories or fat in your diary. (See Part II for more advice regarding which regime or plan to follow).

You can also use your diary to record the following:

- a fat and calorific content list of your favourite/most commonly consumed foods
- graphs detailing your progress

- your motivation to exercise (if your motivation is low, why is this the case)?
- your mood

It's your diary and your aid to success. Use it in a way that helps you.

Measuring Progress

Have you ever heard a person (or yourself) complain about his apparent inability to lose weight despite the fact that he is doing lots of exercise? This is common occurrence and can cause those trying hard to adopt healthier habits to become despondent and return to their old ways. In this example, the person who has been working out regularly and has not appeared to lose any weight *has,* in fact, lost fat and gained muscle mass. Muscle is heavier than fat, so stepping on the scales will not show an expected weight loss in this instance. However, this individual will find that his clothes will feel looser and if he were to measure his hips, waist, chest, thighs and upper arms, he will notice that all measurements have reduced.

This example demonstrates that weight loss is not necessarily an easy thing to measure. As suggested, if you are reducing the amount of calories and fat you are consuming each day in an attempt to lose weight, you may find that if you are exercising (particularly weight training), you may not always appear to lose weight. This section will discuss some of the factors that should be considered whilst trying to monitor your progress. I suggest that you read about all of the different factors and focus on one or two of them as a means of monitoring your progress. (However, constantly bear in mind the other factors, too).

Pounds/Kilograms

(See Appendix 1 for progress table and graph)

It is relatively easy to monitor progress by stepping on scales and noticing the changes in the readings. There are, however, a few things to consider.

- Time of the Day—Always weigh yourself at the same time of the day, wearing the same or similar clothing. Your body weight fluctuates during the day and you may misinterpret a particular reading if taken at a different time of day than your usual practise. I normally find that morning is best.
- Scales—Use the same scales at all times. Different scales give different readings—that's a fact! Sticking to your own familiar scales will give you a more accurate account of your progress. Digital scales are more accurate than your traditional bathroom scales that have a needle. If, however, you're like me, you may prefer to rely on the traditional scales to monitor

your progress. There's something quite satisfying about seeing that needle shift down and down!

- Local Climate—living in a warmer climate may cause you to retain water, which will cause you to put on or not lose weight. Don't worry, it's only fluid and your return to a cooler climate will see that excess fluid get flushed down the pan! (If you live in a warmer climate all year, you may simply notice seasonal changes to your weight as you retain less fluid during the winter months).

- Menstrual Cycle—Ladies, I suspect that most of you know that just as warmer weather can cause you to retain fluid, so too can your period. You'll find that in the days preceding your period, you'll feel bloated, which will be due to retained fluid. This unfortunately will be reflected on the scales. However, once your period has started (or as soon as it's finished), you'll lose this excess fluid.

How much can I expect to lose?

You should generally expect to lose between 2-3kg per month. This will vary, depending on how much weight you want to lose to start with. The more weight you have to lose, the quicker it will seem to come off initially. Most people, regardless of their starting weight, will find that their first month of a new regime will see the biggest weight loss.

How often should I weigh myself?

Don't weigh yourself every day; once a week will suffice. Weighing yourself daily is a bad practise to get into because you can become obsessive and can also be influenced by apparent weight changes that are out with your control (as discussed above). It's not necessary and isn't going to make you lose weight quicker, so don't do it.

What is BMI?

BMI stands for body mass index. It is a calculation that considers both your body mass (weight) and height. It can be calculated by using the formulae below.

BMI = weight (in kg) divided by height (in metres) squared

e.g., If a person is 68 kg and 1.5 m tall, his BMI can be calculated accordingly:

$$BMI = \frac{68}{(1.5)^2}$$

$$= \frac{68}{2.25}$$

$$= 30.2$$

The resultant value is then interpreted in the following way.

BMI above 40	Morbidly Obese
BMI 30-39.9	Obese
BMI 25-29.9	Overweight
BMI 18.5-24.9	Healthy/Normal Weight
BMI less than 18.5	Underweight

Because it is generally recognised that the taller a person is, the heavier he will be compared to a smaller person (assuming that both individuals are of a healthy, normal weight), BMI has been considered to be a more reliable method of assessing whether or not an individual is overweight or underweight than simply measuring weight alone.

However, considering the fact that muscle is heavier than fat, BMI can sometimes be misleading. Consider, for example, an individual who is a body builder; this person may have a BMI of 30. On looking at the table above, it would appear that this individual is considered to be obese, yet it is obvious that this individual's 'excess' body weight is attributed to the high percentage of muscle that he has and not due to a high percentage of fat. As a health professional, I can recall feeling infuriated at the emphasis that one particular nurse put on BMI for providing the most accurate measurement as to whether or not a person was of normal weight or overweight. Before I started my first job as a podiatrist in Glasgow, I was required to undergo a medical assessment. At that particular time, I practised karate (I was almost black belt) and weight trained; I was very fit and had toned muscles. Although my weight was heavier than I would have liked, I tried not to worry about it, reassuring myself that it was largely due to my training regime. This sensible attitude did, however, require a lot of hard work because I was still very sensitive and self-conscious about my image and food-related issues. The occupational health nurse, who undertook my medical history, expressed concern at the fact that my BMI suggested that I was overweight. When I protested, informing her of my weekly exercise regime and reminding her that muscle weighed more than fat, she refused to listen and simply reminded me that the BMI indicated that I was 'overweight'. I went home feeling very upset. (However, on another occasion, when my BMI indicated that I was obese and then morbidly obese, I didn't dispute this because I was). Although many of you reading this will not be unjustly diagnosed as being overweight or obese, you must be aware of the fact that discrepancies can occur and that one should, as previously suggested, consider not only BMI but other factors in order to monitor progress efficiently.

Waist-Hip Ratio & Other Measurements

(See Appendix 2 for progress table)

Science suggests that healthy individuals should have a waist-to-hip ratio of less than 0.85 for women and 1.0 for men. To calculate this ratio, you must divide your waist measurement (taken at the height of your belly button) by your hip measurement (taken at your widest point).

$$\text{Waist-Hip Ratio} = \frac{\underline{Waist\ Measurement}}{Hip\ Measurement}$$

Your waist measurement alone is a key indicator of your health. For optimum health, a woman should have a waist measurement less than 80cm and men 94cm for optimum health. If a woman has a waist measurement of over 88cm and a man over 102cm then she or he is at an increased risk of developing coronary heart disease.

Leading organisations such as the British Heart Foundation state that a person who carries excess fat around their middle (the waist and tummy area)—as opposed to their chest, bottom, thighs or other areas—and have an 'apple' shape have an increased risk of suffering from heart disease. Monitoring a reduction in inches around your waist is therefore an important part of motivating yourself to improve your health.

Likewise, weekly measuring and monitoring the circumference of your thighs, upper arms, bottom, chest, hips, and waist is an excellent way to assess progress—particularly if you are doing cardiovascular exercise and weight training and are developing muscle. Even though your progress (the fact that you're toning up) may not be evident on the scales, you can feel a sense of satisfaction knowing that your measurements are coming down and that your body is becoming healthier.

Frame Size

You may wonder why it is that when you look at literature that indicates what your 'ideal weight' should be, there appears to be a significant range (sometimes as large as 12kg) between which you are considered to be healthy. For example, an individual like me, who is 157cm, is considered healthy anywhere between 49 kg and 60 kg. Prior to my understanding as to why this range existed, I always thought it best just to aim for a weight that was about halfway between the range. Whilst this is not a bad thing to do, an understanding of what category of frame size you have, can help you to aim for a weight that is healthiest for you. All you have to do is measure your wrist then consult the table below which will help you to determine what type of frame size you have and what your ideal healthy weight should be.

<u>*Women*</u>

Height: Under 158cm
- Wrist less than 14 cm = *Small* Frame
- Wrist 14 cm-15 cm = *Medium* Frame
- Wrist greater than 15 cm = *Large* Frame

Height: 158-165cm
- Wrist less than 15 cm = *Small* Frame
- Wrist 15 cm-16 cm = *Medium* Frame
- Wrist greater than 16 cm = *Large* Frame

Height: Over 165cm
- Wrist less than 16 cm = *Small* Frame
- Wrist 16 cm-17 cm = *Medium* Frame
- Wrist greater than 17 cm = *Large* Frame

<u>*Men*</u>

Height: Under 165cm
- Wrist less than 16 cm = *Small* Frame
- Wrist 16 cm-17 cm = *Medium* Frame
- Wrist greater than 17 cm = *Large* Frame

Height: Over 165cm
- Wrist less than 17 cm = *Small* Frame
- Wrist 17 cm-19 cm = *Medium* Frame
- Wrist greater than 19 cm = *Large* Frame

Body Fat Percentage

Body fat percentage is a measure of the amount of fat as opposed to lean tissue that contributes to the overall mass of an individual. It provides a more accurate indication of health than measuring weight alone because, as previously discussed, muscle is heavier than fat. Two individuals who are of the same height may be different sizes but may weigh the same; the individual who wears the smaller sized clothes will be more toned and have more muscle, but he will weigh the same as the person who wears the larger clothes, because muscle weighs more than fat.

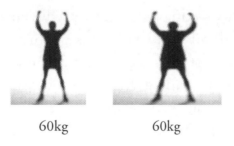

60kg   60kg

Many bathroom scales are now capable of measuring both mass and body fat percentage. A body fat percentage is obtained once a miniscule electric current is passed through the body. Lean tissue conducts electricity and fat doesn't, so a differentiation is made between the two and an overall percentage of body fat can therefore be determined. Generally speaking, it is recognised that for women a body fat percentage of between 25-31 per cent is acceptable and for men it is 18-25 per cent. Variations exist when age is considered; younger adults (in their early twenties) should have a smaller percentage of body fat and older individuals (over fifty) should have a higher percentage of body fat. If you are uncertain as to what is healthy for you, please consult a health professional.

Other Factors to Consider

Besides the different ways in which progress may be monitored, there are other factors that one must consider which may influence both perceived and actual weight loss. Such factors include the following.

- Activity—Although exercise will be discussed in more detail in 'Part II', it is worth noting that the inclusion of physical activity into one's routine will obviously speed up the process of weight loss (as well as benefiting one's health in other ways).
- Clothing—The significance of clothing should not be overlooked. Not only can your clothing indicate (by feeling loose or tight) how much or little progress you are making, but it can also influence your emotional state (including how confident you feel). I'm sure that most people can relate to that good feeling they experience when they wear clothing that suits their shape, fits them properly and is a colour that complements their hair, eyes and skin colour. All of us deserve to experience that good feeling every day! If you are losing weight, you must aim to feel the

best you can. Show love and respect for yourself by rewarding your efforts and wearing these 'feel good' clothes every day. If you are losing weight, be careful that you don't wear clothes that are too big because this can actually make you look heavier than you actually are and be demotivating. If you are losing weight steadily and are struggling to keep up with the need to purchase smaller sizes of clothing, you may need to limit your wardrobe to a few essential items that can be worn as day, evening, or work wear. If money is tight, as it was for me, you may wish to buy second-hand clothes from a charity shop. (I would always purchase such clothing from charity shops that were situated in the more affluent parts of the city. I found that there was better quality garments in these shops).

- Compliments—When the compliments on your weight loss start to roll in, you know you're on the right track! Some people will notice your achievements quicker than others. The person who will be the first to notice your success is you! Make sure you remember to congratulate yourself! You deserve all the praise you can get, but do remember to stay focussed and on track until you get to your target weight. Remember to reward yourself with non-food treats. Ask yourself what you would really appreciate, make a list, and stick it onto your fridge. My list of rewards included the following:

o going to the cinema (to which I'd take an apple and drink a low-calorie drink)
o buying some flowers
o going for a walk in the park and appreciating the beauty of nature
o going for a facial
o getting my hair cut
o painting my nails
o having a bath with bubbles

If you find that the complements are taking their time to come your way, be patient—it won't be long before they start and once they do, if you remain on track, they will not stop! When this happens, I can tell you, it feels great!

- Mirrors and Photos—Mirrors are obviously a useful way to help reveal your progress, but just be mindful of the fact that different mirrors can make you appear larger or smaller. Also, sometimes you may be too critical and see yourself as being bigger than you actually are, or you may see yourself as being smaller than you are. (This can happen if you are at the start of your new regime and are maybe in denial as to how big you really are). I have experienced both illusions and now tend to take a more holistic view when monitoring my health (i.e., how my clothes feel, how *I* feel). Something that I have noticed is that I always seem to get a 'true' representation as to what I look like in photographs. You may therefore start to take photos of yourself on a regular basis. (If you are camera shy, don't worry; as you lose weight, you will find that your shyness will become a thing of the past. You will discover that you actually *want* to get your photograph taken)!

What Is a Balanced Diet?

Low fat, no fat, no trans fats, sugar-free, low GI, low sugar, complex carbs . . . What does it all mean? Eating a 'healthy' diet can become really complicated if you allow it to become so, but that doesn't have to be the case; this will be explained later. First I want to tell you about different foods that are out there.

Carbohydrates

Carbohydrates are any food that contains some form of sugar, which is broken down to provide energy. Often dieters attempt to cut the carbs, deeming them to be 'bad', but this is not necessarily the case. As far as carbohydrates are concerned, different types exist.

- **Simple Carbohydrates**—These are foods that contain 1-2 units of sugar and include cakes, white bread and generally speaking foodstuffs that contain table sugar. These are often referred to as being the 'bad' carbohydrates.

- **Complex Carbohydrates**—These are starchy foods and are mostly essential for a balanced diet. They include brown bread, grains, brown rice, wholemeal pasta and more. They are an excellent source of fibre—something that makes you feel full. Some complex carbohydrates release energy more slowly than others. For good health, you should try to eat complex carbohydrates that release energy slowly (e.g., oats and pulses). The slow release in energy means that you will not experience a slump in energy shortly after eating them, as you would do with other foods.

Fruits and Vegetables

The benefits of eating fruits and vegetables are numerous. This food group should make up at least one-third of your daily diet. If you're reading this and thinking, 'But I don't even know what an apple looks like,' please, do not be put off by what you have read. Eating a diet that is comprised mainly of fruits and vegetables is not something that will happen overnight. Any new regime requires patience and often one needs to take small steps before it becomes a habit and doesn't feel like a chore.

The British Heart Foundation, along with other reputable agencies and advisory boards, advises the public to eat five portions of fruit and/or vegetables a a day. Many individuals, however, are unclear as to what five portions actually is and other countries actually advise people to eat seven or eight portions of fruit and vegetables a day. There is also confusion as to what fruits and vegetables should be eaten. Quite simply, one should not drink five glasses of supermarket 'freshly squeezed juice' and consider oneself to have met the recommended 'five a day' nor should one only eat fruit (even a variety) in order to meet the quota. As mentioned previously, this food group should eventually constitute much more than five a day of your daily diet and it should contain a *variety* of different types of fruits and vegetables, such as the following:

- *Seasonal Fruits*—different varieties of locally grown fruits can be in abundance at different times in the year. They tend to be at their tastiest and cheapest when they are in season.
- *Exotic Fruits*—In the UK these fruits are imported from warmer climates and include mango, pineapple, papaya and more. Although they can sometimes be more expensive, they are a nice treat.
- *Berries*—Blueberries, strawberries, raspberries are so delicious and nutritious! They can be eaten by themselves, can be part of a fruit salad or a smoothie, or added to breakfast cereal or yoghurt.
- *Pure Juice*—Squeeze your own juice at home—that way you'll *know* that it's 100 per cent pure juice and doesn't have any additives.
- *Vegetables*—Aim to have a variety of colours and eat different vegetables because they all have different (very powerful) nutritional benefits (including anti-cancer and anti-aging properties).

- *Soups*—Soups are an excellent way to include vegetables into your diet, especially if you have not yet developed a passionate desire to consume them (this will happen, though)! You can add pulses to soups; not only will these bulk the soup up and make you feel fuller, but they also contain a rich source of nutrients such as calcium, magnesium and folic acid, to name a few.
- *Salads*—Salads can taste great, especially if you are prepared to be a bit more adventurous and add fruits, vegetables, nuts, seeds and a small portion of cheese.

Fruits and vegetables should form the backbone of one's daily diet. However, in order to gain the maximum amount of nutrition from fruit and vegetables, you should eat them in their purest form—that is, uncooked and without the addition of any sauces, sugar, or cream. With that said, I believe that in order to maintain a healthy eating regime that will see you through until the day you die, you have to be realistic but also have an awareness of what you are eating. For example, if you have enjoyed a rich source of uncooked, raw fruit and vegetables during most of the day and you are cooking dinner for your family and friends in the evening, it is perfectly acceptable to give your guests a salad that has a small amount of low-fat dressing added to it. Alternatively, you may decide to cook a vegetable stew and for dessert you can have a chocolate banana cake—homemade, using the healthiest possible ingredients, of course! At the end of the day, food is there to be enjoyed; that is why we have been blessed with taste buds! As well as making the sharing and tasting of food enjoyable, you should aim to make it as healthy as possible (just remember, if it tastes bland, it will not be enjoyable). I cannot stress the enjoyment element enough—this is because we all know that we do not stick with anything that we do not enjoy.

You may come across advice that conflicts with what I have advised regarding bulking your daily diet with fruit and vegetables. Many experts are divided as far as this is concerned. Many food pyramids (figure 1) can be seen as having a bottom group (i.e., what should constitute the largest food group in a daily diet) that consists of complex carbohydrates. On the other hand, many diet plates (figure 2), will depict equal sized complex carbohydrates and fruit and vegetable portions, suggesting that equal quantities of both groups should be consumed.

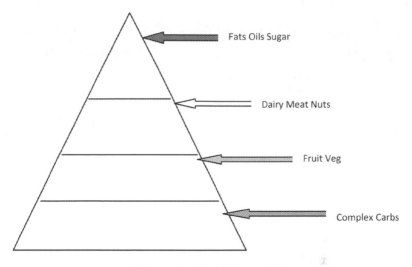

Figure 1—Food Pyramid

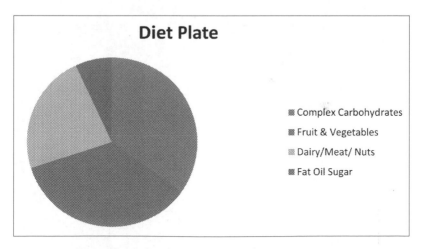

Figure 2 Diet Plate

The differences in advice and information offered therefore call for the health-conscious person to make their own decisions. Just bear in mind what I mentioned about different countries advising different daily quantities of fruits and vegetables and you may feel a little more qualified to do this! Whatever you do, you should aim to

- have a *minimum* of five portions of fruits and vegetables every day and
- try to keep your diet as 'pure' (unprocessed) as possible.

If in doubt, seek out professional advice from a qualified and registered dietician. Your family doctor can refer you if you ask. (See *Part III 'Other Information, Advice & Support').*

PART II

What's Right for Me?

Okay, so you know that you want to, need to and are ready to change. You've got all your information at your fingertips and you know that there are things that you can do or not do that will make this easier.

The trouble is, you have been given so much advice and so many recommendations that you just don't know what's right for you. Just as we all have different journeys through life that are unique and significant; our weight-loss journeys are unique and should be treated as such. By all means, listen to the advice and suggestions given to you by different people. As you accumulate more knowledge, you will be able to quickly identify what advice is worth adhering to and what advice deserves to be flushed down the toilet!

I will offer some healthy suggestions in this section of the book that will help you to decide how to go about achieving your goal. I encourage you to read this section in its entirety, writing notes in the margin as required and consider what path or paths you are going to follow that complement *your* lifestyle and are right for *you.*

Motivation & Social Situations

Before I discuss the specific elements that are obviously essential to any weight loss regime, I would like to discuss tactics and issues that require mental training and development. The development of such tactics and an understanding of the issues at hand must not be overlooked.

Motivation

You *must* build your armour. At first, you will feel really motivated, but believe me that motivation will diminish, sometimes quickly. The question is, how do you keep your motivation alive? The answer, in part, is that you have to build your armour to keep it alive even *before* you embark on a new, healthier journey. You can try to adopt all or some of these strategies.

- *Buy health magazines* like *Top Sante* and *Zest* (Later, you may wish to purchase magazines that are more specific to sports that you may, and probably will, become passionate about).

- *Try not to socialise with people who have poor eating habits or who may ridicule your attempts to improve your health.* Often such people will want you to eat

unhealthy or unplanned for food, simply to keep them company whilst they indulge and to make them feel less guilty. If unkind or unfair comments are made, try to remind yourself that unkind comments tend to be made by individuals who are either jealous or feel threatened in some way. Do not respond to such comments—instead, congratulate yourself for doing well. Whatever you do, do not preach to an overweight friend about the importance of healthy eating; other people will resent you for this. Instead, lead by example. I found that by keeping my diet a secret, I was able to minimise negative comments and inspired people because they could *see* the results.

- *Visualise yourself as being at your goal weight.* I know that this sounds crazy, but it *does* work. Imagine yourself at your ideal weight, wearing the clothes that you really want to wear and feeling the emotions that you know you really want and deserve to feel— they are trapped inside you! Go on and fantasize, make your image real! Imagine where you are and walk around your image, viewing yourself from every angle. Imagine how your clothes feel to touch, how your hair looks, how you feel, and what complements you can hear coming your way. Do this and then capture this image and store it in your head; before you go to sleep at night, revisit it. Do this *every* night. I promise you, it works!

Those people who are closest to me and whom I love very much say that I am into 'mumbo jumbo'! Well, I have tried to tell them that my mumbo jumbo—or hypnotherapy, visualizations and positive affirmations—*does* work! I came across it quite by accident. Like many others, I had been looking for a tool or trick that would help me on my mission to lose weight. I came across a self-help slimming tape in my local bookstore. I purchased the tape, not really believing it would help but wanting to believe. I listened to it a couple of times and then put it in the back of my drawer because it didn't give me the instant 'cure' I was craving.

About two years later, when I had reached a crossroads and knew that I either had to lose weight or die, I decided that I would listen to the tape again, every night, as instructed, in an attempt to *help* me. This time, my expectations had changed; I knew that there was no instant cure for my weight loss and that at the end of the day, any tools or tricks were only there to help me and not to do the work for me. Not dismissing the power of any help I could get, I decided to follow the instructions given to me on the tape to the letter. The instructions were quite simple: listen to the tape every night before going to sleep. So *every* night, for at least eight months, I listened to my tape and envisaged myself at my ideal weight.

It was only at my uncle's wedding, which occurred at the tenth month of my weight loss journey, that I realised my visualizations had in fact become a reality! For eight months I had envisaged myself wearing a pair of black pin-striped trousers with a black long-sleeved top with a brooch. Guess what I wore to the wedding? You've guessed it! This was done unconsciously since I had at that time not listened to my tape in well over a month, and I did not even consider my visual image when choosing my wedding clothes.

I am not suggesting that you have to rush out and buy a hypnotherapy CD, because all that the guy on the tape told me to do was exactly what I've advised you to do—visualize yourself at your target weight, actually put yourself *in* the ideal you and experience how it feels. It's great, isn't it! I know that it works because not only did I apply this to my weight loss regime, but I also started to visualize myself being accepted into a post-graduate university course (which I had been unsuccessful in qualifying for before) and passing my driving test (which I had previously failed four times). So in the same year, thanks to visualization, believing in myself, positive thinking (or positive affirmations), and not giving up, I managed to pass my driving test, lose a staggering amount of weight, and get accepted into a highly competitive post-graduate course. What a year! It really did reinforce the power that these mental exercises had. Your mind is a powerful tool that you can use to your advantage.

• Something you can do that ties in with visualization is the use of pictures. Cut out either pictures of yourself when you were slimmer and at an ideal weight, or pictures of other thinner people whom you aspire to look like. (If you have pictures of other people, stick a picture of your face on top of the other person's face). Then attach the pictures on to your fridge or a vision board. A vision board is a poster that has pictures of all your goals and dreams. It is another very powerful tool. Keeping pictures on your fridge is a good idea because this is where much of your food will be kept! Some people like to put 'fat' pictures on display—that is, photographs showing themselves at their heaviest weight. I personally find this to be unhelpful because it just serves to trigger unhappy feelings and reminds you of what you were. Whatever you focus on, you tend to get more of, so if you continue to focus on the fat picture on the fridge, the chances are you will just remain fat. This activity is therefore not motivating— it is demotivating.

I would love to say that it has all been plain sailing since I reached my target weight, but it hasn't. There are times when I do go back to my old ways and over-indulge if I've had a 'bad day', but I never underestimate the power that self-hypnosis, visualizations and positive thinking has. I practise these strategies on a regular basis because they help me to remain focussed and positive. It is encouraging to notice that as I continue to practise these strategies and my mental armour gets stronger and stronger, I seem to be less disturbed by the so-called stresses in life and have fewer and fewer 'bad' days. It is both fascinating and exciting to witness my development. I encourage you to give it a try!

I have hinted at the fact that losing weight is not easy. Well, now I want to say this more clearly: this is *not* going to be easy. However, it *does not* have to be a struggle, and it *will* get easier.

However you decide to start, you need to have a plan. You need to do all of the reflective exercises mentioned at the start of this book and then you need to stick with whatever rules and boundaries that you have created for yourself. You will probably find that the first three to five days of your new diet regime may be quite challenging as far as the food aspect is concerned. During this period, you will have to be strong and constantly remind yourself how disappointed you will feel if you don't stick to your plan. You may find it helpful to keep a small supply of healthy food in your bag so that if you are tempted to reach for the chocolate or other favoured unhealthy foods, you can say to yourself, 'I know I think I want XYZ, but I am not going to waste any money or damage myself by having it. Instead, I will have the healthy snack in my bag. If I am truly hungry, the snack will help to satisfy my hunger.' The formation of this new habit does require a lot of discipline at first, but eventually you will find yourself opting for the healthier options without any conscious effort or need of willpower.

Remember at all times to praise yourself. Other people may not notice any weight loss to start with, nor will they know what goals you have set yourself on a day-to-day basis. The praise of other people will eventually flow in abundance towards you, but until it does, it is vital that your efforts are praised by your best friend—yourself! If you know that you have managed to get through a particularly challenging week, then praise and treat yourself with a non-food treat. You can refer to your list of treats that you compiled earlier.

Social Situations

Social situations can present their own challenges and can prove difficult, but only if you let them. Although you must have awareness and exercise control as far as your diet is concerned, there is no reason why you should deprive yourself from having a good time. The key is to be prepared and to acknowledge the fact that food and drink (including alcohol) are not the only sources of pleasure.

If you are at the initial stages of your journey, you may have to be more choosey about which situations you involve yourself. I have suggested this because you may be more likely to succumb to temptation at this stage. Other times when you may be likely to give in to temptation include the following:

- times of stress, frustration, anxiety, feeling down, or any other negative emotion
- times of tiredness
- feelings of elation and extreme happiness
- pre-menstruation

If you are organised and plan ahead for such times, then you should be able to get through these times with minimum disruption to your healthy eating regime. For example, if you have been invited to a party that, you have been told, will not finish until the early hours of the morning, then you must carefully plan your diet before, during, and after the party. Eating lower calorie and lower fat foods during the day before the party will allow you a bit of flexibility to indulge a little at the party. Drinking plenty of water before the party will not only fill you up but will also help your body to cope with any alcohol consumed.

Prior to the party, you should set a limit as to how many alcoholic drinks you have. Try to avoid alco-pops, beer and cream-based liqueurs. Obviously if such drinks are your preferred choice, then enjoy one, but then switch to red or dry white wine or spirits mixed with a low-calorie mixer. Try to anticipate what food will be served at the function and plan what you will eat. If you are going to a buffet, look at all of the food first, decide what you would like to eat, then fill up your dinner plate with a little bit of what you want, ensuring that you include vegetables and salad. Once you have put the food on your plate that you want and feel that you can eat without over-indulging, sit back down, enjoy your main course and eat it slowly. Do not go back up for second or third helpings. Decide beforehand whether you will opt for a starter or a dessert and limit yourself to a smaller portion of your chosen course. You could even share a starter or a dessert. If you are in a restaurant and choosing from a menu, ask for a smaller portion (including children's portions) or find out if it is possible to have a starter as a main course. An increasing number of restaurants are used to dealing with such requests, so don't be shy to ask.

Ensure that you continue to drink lots of water during and after a party. If you have consumed alcohol during the party, you will find that your resistance to unhealthy junk food is lower. Be prepared! Have some brown bread at home, so that when the party is over and you are back home feeling hungry, you can make yourself some wholemeal toast rather than calling for the delivery pizza. Have healthy foods on hand for the following day; aim to fill yourself up with healthy fruit and cereal first and only then, if you are still craving some greasy or sweet food, allow yourself to indulge *a little*. Chances are you will find that your healthy food has left you feeling full and satisfied, so your urge to indulge in junk food will diminish. To avoid this situation and a hangover, do what I often do and take the car (knowing, of course that I can't consume any alcohol since it is illegal to drink and drive).

If you have been invited to a friend's house for a less formal occasion and you know that your friend is going to order take-away for everyone, plan ahead by bringing your own food! Yes, it may seem a little inappropriate and you may feel awkward, but at the end of the day, your health comes first. Whilst we all know that the extra calories and fat consumed during one night off will not cause you to regain your lost weight, the one night off may have damaging mental consequences in that it could cause you to fall off the wagon and ditch the diet completely. You must therefore be strong, be prepared, and don't be shy to act in the name of health! In this situation, you could ease any awkwardness that you feel by cooking or buying lots of healthy food that you can share with everyone.

Don't be afraid to say no if you are offered something to eat. Some people, however, can be very pushy though they often have good intentions, and they can practically force food onto you. If this happens and you know that the word no will just cause insult or hassle that you would rather avoid, accept a small piece of the food offered and either eat it very slowly (talking a lot in between mouthfuls is a good strategy), or don't eat it at all (instead, just push it around your plate with your fork and 'lose' your plate of food once your host has left you). If you know that you really cannot risk accepting any food, pretend that you are ill or have just eaten. I know that these measures sound extreme, but I also know that many people simply do not understand how much strength and motivation is required (especially at the initial stages) by an individual who has decided to embark on a healthy eating regime. You are doing what is right for you and if other people make discouraging comments, you must remind yourself that your health and happiness comes first.

If you do find that your night out has caused you to completely overindulge, *don't* use this as an excuse to give up. Instead, reflect on why you chose to overeat and think about what you could do to avoid a repeat of this incident. For example, if, in the future, you are invited to a social event and deep down you know that going to the event will cause you to overindulge, it may be worthwhile asking yourself if it is really worth going it at all. You strongly suspect that you will eat too much; how will you feel afterwards? If your cravings for junk food are particularly strong at this time, it may be worthwhile reaching a kind of compromise in your head. For example, if I felt like this, I would avoid the particular social situation if I could and indulge my craving by making or buying a healthier alternative. Then, in an attempt to not be anti-social, I would arrange to meet my friends for a coffee (and perhaps explain my dilemma, if appropriate). The avoidance of parties and other social activities is not something that I would condone, however there were two or three occasions when I had to put into practise what I have just advised. On these occasions, I know that going to the functions would have meant disaster for my regime.

If you are going out for a day, make sure you have a healthy snack in your bag. Always eat your healthy snack first before going to a cafe or restaurant. If you are eating out, ask to look at a menu before you order. (You may be surprised to find that some coffee shops are cafes offer healthier snacks).

Exercise

'Ouch! No thanks!' I bet many of you are thinking such thoughts. Well, to all of you who feel this way, I challenge you to ask yourself, 'What if exercise might not actually be the unpleasant thing that I think it is?' Even if you're not convinced that the answer is, 'Well, it's not that unpleasant,' I challenge you to at least give it a serious go to find out. Surely all these exercise freaks can't all be lying when they say that they actually enjoy exercise.

One of the things that made me feel less intimidated by exercise was the realisation that exercise is in fact any activity that involves moving. Something as simple as walking constitutes as exercise. At this time in my life, the thought of walking was even too tiring for my brain, but the realisation of the fact that exercise helps to burn fat made me seriously rethink my attitude towards the whole thing. My ultimate goal was to be thinner and healthier and I wanted to achieve my goal at the fastest (and healthiest) pace possible. I kept thinking about those 'normal' clothes shops and dare I even say it, skinny jeans and knee-high boots! However, before you reach for your walking shoes, I want you to consider the following.

- When you are starting out, don't include exercise in your new healthier regime if you don't want to. If you know that you really need to focus on your diet alone, then do this. After your new eating habits are second nature, you can think about exercise.
- Only do exercise that you enjoy. At first, no exercise may appeal to you. If this is the case, you must engage in an activity that is the least intimidating and can be done alone or in a group and at a preferred location (e.g., walking).
- Wear clothing and footwear which is comfortable and sensible. Wear lace-up shoes and weather-appropriate clothing (e.g., waterproofs, warm clothing, lightweight cool clothing, etc.). You will not stick with your activity if you do not wear appropriate clothing. Who cares what you look like—you are doing this for your health! Ladies, remember to wear a supportive sports bra; besides allowing you to feel more comfortable, a quality sports bra will reduce any movement of and therefore help to protect your breasts. Try to get your bra fitted by a shop attendant who is trained to do so, because it is extremely important that you wear the correct size of bra.
- Try listening to music whilst you exercise alone. I put a lot of disco and happy music on my iPod. I find that it really spurs me on!
- Give yourself small goals. Write up a two-week or four-week schedule. Try to increase either the time or intensity of your workouts slowly. For example, let's

say you started walking for ten minutes during your exercise sessions in your first week. So long as you felt comfortably challenged doing this, you could then either increase your activity to twelve minutes the second week, or stick with ten minutes and change your route to one which involves some small hills. The temptation would be to increase the time *and* the intensity, or to increase the time to more than twelve minutes (say, to fifteen minutes). Well, *don't*. You will burn yourself out, lose motivation and not stick with it. At the end of the day, you want to follow a regime that you will stick to, don't you?

- Have rest days to start with and aim to exercise no more than three times a week. After a month, you can increase this to four or five times a week, but don't do any more than this. Your body needs to rest (even if it is only walking that you choose to do).

- After a month of doing your chosen exercises, you must aim to weight train at least twice a week. Lifting weights will not only help to tone your muscles, but it will also help you to burn fat even when you are resting because your metabolism will increase (fancy that!) and it will help to strengthen your bones, protecting against osteoporosis (women especially). If the thought of going to a gym scares you, try it; if you're female, go to a ladies gym. Go to a Local Authority gym (these gyms tend to attract all different shapes and sizes), or call your preferred gym to find out when their quiet time is. If you are *really* opposed to visiting a gym, you can attempt to exercise at home by following a fitness DVD. A word of caution though: if you are determined to exercise at home, you will have to be *very* disciplined.

- If you've enrolled in a class but never go, you can't say that you do this particular activity. The fact that you never go suggests that it probably is either not an activity that motivates you, or is not on at a time or day of the week which most suits you. I am one of these people who likes to exercise before I go to work. Some people think that I'm crazy, but it suits me. I have tried exercising in the evening, to avoid having to go to bed quite so early, but it really doesn't work for me. I find that I get lazy and just don't do the same intensity of exercise as I do in the morning. You must find a time of day and an activity that suits you, because it's your life, your health and your happiness that's important. If we don't do what's right for us, we won't stick with whatever it is we're forcing ourselves to do. It's taken years for me to discover that!

What Diet Should I Follow?

Choosing a diet can be the really confusing bit because there are so many out there. What you have to do is to bear in mind that your diet should actually resemble a healthy eating plan and not just offer a solution to weight loss. You want to follow a diet that adheres to the advice given in the food pyramid or diet plate (as previously shown). Therefore, most of your daily consumption should be made up of fruit and vegetables and complex carbohydrates. Do not be tempted to follow a diet (or detox) which eliminates any of the food groups. You may seem to lose weight, but chances are it will be fluid and not fat you are losing. Such diets are not sustainable because they are limiting and often socially isolating, which results in demotivation and failure to achieve your goal. Even if your diet does promote fat loss, you will not stick to it and eventually will put back on all the weight you have lost!

Like most people, you will want to lose the weight fast, but I must tell you that *there is no quick-fix solution to weight loss*. It takes time and does require patience and determination, but once you've reached your goal, you will feel so proud of yourself! Try not to let the idea that it takes time put you off from starting—you have to start at some point, don't you? Why let twelve months pass when you could have reached your target weight by that point? Surely it's better to start your journey now rather than procrastinate and put it off. That said, if you find that you are really not in the right frame of mind to start right now, try to sort out the clutter in your mind that's holding you back and set a date in the next six weeks when you plan to start.

Slimming Clubs

Joining a slimming club is a great way to get motivation and support. Depending on which club you join, you will receive advice as to how much and what you should be eating.

Clubs like Weight Watchers have Internet memberships for those people who can't attend a weekly meeting. They also offer a great selection of menus and recipes that can be used at home. Weight Watchers, in particular, tends to have a sensible and healthy approach, which is why I've referred to it. I'm sure that there are other clubs which offer healthy advice and with which I am not familiar. So long as the club that you choose to go to advocates a healthy diet that resembles the food pyramid or diet plate and includes all food groups, you will be fine.

Professional Advice

There are many different professionals who can offer valuable advice, if you require it. A good starting point in seeking advice is to visit your family doctor. Most clinics have nurses who can offer advice, and some even have a dietician who can give you specific information and guidance to help you make healthier choices. Some clinics offer weekly 'healthy living' or 'weight loss' classes that offer advice, encouragement and the opportunity to have your weight recorded.

If your clinic does not have a dietician, you can speak to your doctor, who may be able to refer you to one provided that he or she considers it to be appropriate for your health needs. Should you or your doctor feel that your weight issues are due to an underlying mental health issue (such as depression or low self-esteem), you may be referred to a psychologist or a mental health nurse.

If you do seek help and are offered it, accept it willingly and take on board the advice that you are given. If you are already familiar with some of the advice and information that you are given, do not dismiss it as being old news. Instead, be grateful for the chance to reconsider and revise what you already know! If you find that you have a negative attitude towards any advice or professional who is giving advice, it may be that you are not ready to lose weight and must reconsider your motives for embarking on this journey. If you find that you are not ready, don't worry—you will just have to wait until you are!

A hypnotherapist may be able to help you to visualize yourself at your target weight. The support that a hypnotherapist can offer complements what I have suggested earlier: if you believe that your goal is already a reality, then it will very likely become a reality. What you think about or focus on becomes a reality.

A life coach can also help you achieve your goal. I visited a life coach whilst I was working in Saudi Arabia. I had a few goals that I wanted to achieve (including writing this book), yet procrastination and 'other stuff' seemed to be get in the way. My life coach made me realise which of my goals I *really* did want to achieve and understand why I hadn't managed to be proactive up until that point. I also understood that my goals would not become a reality unless I acted. Without action, nothing would change.

Going Alone

Only embark on this journey alone if you are confident that you will not fall off the wagon or lose sight of what your ultimate goal is—that is, to eat a healthy diet (as well as to lose weight). You should also only go alone if you have a thorough understanding of the following.

- what your nutritional needs are
- how much weight you should expect to lose
- what your ideal weight should be
- how many calories or how much fat you should be consuming at every stage of your journey

Although I embarked on my journey alone, it is worth remembering that I am a qualified health professional and after the first month of my journey, I encouraged my friend to lose weight too. She was staying in my spare room at the time, which was a real benefit to both of us. We both spurred each other on and because we knew that we'd feel guilty if the other one saw us eating something unhealthy or unplanned, we just didn't! I'm glad to say that both of us reached our target weight at a healthy rate.

If you are in any doubt as to what you should be doing, or if after a month of going alone, you find that you have not made any progress, then go and join a slimming club or get support from a health professional.

If you do decide to go alone, you need to decide whether or not you should focus on a fat-controlled diet or a calorie-controlled diet.

Fat

If you prefer to limit your daily fat consumption, you must familiarise yourself with the different types of fat.

There are several different types of fat. Many people perceive all fat as being bad, but this is not the case. Whilst some fats should be avoided or consumed in small quantities, there are other fats that are essential for health. The table below details the different names and qualities of different fats that are present in every day foods.

Saturated Fat	This is the worst type of fat since it poses the greatest risk to health. It can be found in meat, dairy produce, crisps and sweets. Saturated fat can be easily identified since it turns white when it solidifies. It should be eaten in moderation.
Polyunsaturated Fat	This is not as dense as saturated fat and is actually beneficial to health. Omega 3 is a type of polyunsaturated fat which can be found in oily fish and actually lowers cholesterol.
Monounsaturated Fat	Monounsaturated fat is also thought to be beneficial to health. It can be found in olive oil, olives, nuts, and avocado pears.
Trans Fats	This is a fat which was polyunsaturated and has had hydrogen added to it to change it into saturated fat. It is highly damaging to health, causing an increase in bad cholesterol and susceptibility to heart disease. Some food companies have stopped adding trans fats to their products, recognising their threat to health. Sometimes the omission of trans fat in a product is clearly displayed on the packaging.

Calories

Calories are another word for energy. The amount of energy (calories) you need obviously varies depending on how much energy you spend (exercise you do). Think of your body as being a car and of calories as being petrol.

The more you drive (exercise), the more petrol (calories) you need.

and

The less driving you do, the less petrol you will need.

If you are trying to shift excess weight, you essentially have to get your body to use the stores of energy it already has (excess fat), rather than use energy from food you may have eaten.

You need to understand how much energy (calories) your body needs in order to do its daily activities, and then eat slightly less than this to ensure that your body starts to burn unwanted fat. The table below will give you an idea as to what your daily energy requirements are.

Sedentary Lifestyle	Moderately Active Lifestyle (exercise 3-4 half-hour sessions per week)	Active Lifestyle
Weight (kg) x 31 = Total number of calories that can be consumed daily (without causing a change in weight)	Weight (kg) x 37 = Total number of calories that can be consumed daily (without causing a change in weight)	Weight (kg) x 44 = Total number of calories that can be consumed daily (without causing a change in weight)

Information obtained from Collins Gem Calorie Counter

As I mentioned in Part I, the figures quoted are influenced by your frame size and also whether or not you are overweight to start with. You can be confident that the figures quoted in the table above will be very close to your specific calorific consumption. If you are 6-12kg overweight, you should use the information above to determine how many calories you will need to carry out your daily activities. For example, let's say Sue is a thirty-year-old woman who is 6kg overweight and does one hour of exercise each week. Sue has a sedentary lifestyle, so she needs to eat 2,100 calories in order to maintain her weight as it is. If Sue wants to gain weight, she must continue to maintain her sedentary lifestyle and eat more calories. If Sue wants to lose weight, she must eat fewer calories and even increase the amount of exercise she does.

If you are losing weight, your body will do this in stages. In each stage, your body will reach a point where it seems incapable of losing any more weight, despite the fact that you are vigilantly continuing to adopt a healthy lifestyle. At the start of your new regime, you need to look at the figure quoted in the table and subtract two hundred calories from that. This should be the number of calories that you will need to consume in order to ensure steady and healthy weight loss. Once you reach the start of a new stage, you will need to subtract another one hundred calories from your daily allowance.

However, do not consume less than 1,400 calories per day if you are a woman, and 1,700 calories per day if you are a man. If you consume less than this, you will cause your metabolism to slow down because your body will believe it is starving. If your metabolism slows down, this means that you will put on weight easily. You will also feel very grumpy and lack energy. If you are down to these minimum figures and are not losing any more weight, it is very likely that you are at your ideal weight—yippee!

Each stage will last for anywhere between three to eight weeks, so if we look at Sue's case, we can see how she had to alter her calorie consumption.

Jan	1900 cals	Size 16
Feb	1800 cals	Size 15
Mid Mar	1700 cals	Size 14
Jun	1600 cals	Size 13
Jul	1500 cals	Size12
Aug	1400 cals	Size10—Target Size!

If Sue was more than 12kg overweight, she may need to start off by eating more calories. This is because the heavier we are, the more energy (calories) needed by our bodies to do our daily activities. I'm sure that many of you will be familiar with ankle weights. Many fitness experts encourage the use of ankle weights because your body has to work harder to carry extra weight, and you effectively burn off unwanted fat at a faster rate. If you are overweight, the same principals apply.

At all times you must listen to your body. Love and respect it. If you are struggling to stick to your daily calorific allowance, then increase it *slightly.* Don't struggle on and regard this as being some kind of unpleasant chore—if you do, you will not remain motivated and will very likely fail to reach your goal.

PART III

Other Information, Advice & Support

Fluids

As you lose weight, you will pass a lot of fluid at the beginning. It can be a bit frustrating to continually have to go to the toilet, but this will only be a temporary problem. I would encourage you to aim to drink 1.5-2 litres of pure water every day. (In hot climates, like the Gulf, where I was working, I had to drink around three litres of water every day. The same applies if you are exercising: you will need more water).

If you are not used to drinking pure water, then by all means try adding some sugar-free juice. Only add a little, though and try to wean yourself off this so that you are eventually drinking only water. Pure water is great for you: it has no fat, calories, or artificial ingredients. It helps you feel full and is essential for your body's general well-being. It makes your eyes, skin and hair look healthy and you will look younger!

If you are a fizzy drink fan, try to cut these out; even if they are sugar free or diet versions, they are so bad for your teeth, bones, and general health. If you like tea and coffee, try to limit this too, since both are diuretics (i.e., they make you pass urine). Many fizzy drinks are also diuretics.

Alcohol can actually contain a lot of calories. As mentioned previously, the consumption of alcohol itself can also stimulate the appetite, weaken your resolve not to eat unhealthy food and cause dehydration. It also disturbs sleep, causing you to feel tired, which again weakens your resolve not to eat unhealthy food. Alcohol also has no nutritional benefits, so if you are trying to limit the number of calories you are consuming, it makes sense to limit the amount of alcohol you consume or abstain from it altogether.

Diet Pills

Here's my advice about diet pills: quite simply put, *don't go there!* Over-the-counter 'herbal' pills are a complete and utter waste of money. If you choose to use them, the only thing you'll lose is money! Herbal pills may be presented in shops with promises to help you lose a certain amount of weight in a given time period. If such tablets really were *the* miracle cure for weight loss, then surely this miracle cure would be widely publicized on the news and in the press. Would doctors surgeries and health stores not be inundated with people desperate to get their hands on this miracle cure?

The same is true for those diet pills that can only be prescribed by a qualified health professional. None of these prescribed drugs offer a miracle cure, either—in fact they can end up giving you more than you bargained for.

Some prescription drugs work by eliminating ingested fat from your system. This means that any fat consumed is simply passed through your body in the form of an orange-coloured fluid similar to cooking oil. Elimination of fat can occur unexpectedly and without a patient even being aware of its passing out of their body! This can cause much embarrassment because clothing and furnishings can end up being stained bright orange. If you are taking these pills, use of a sanitary towel (by both men and women) is highly recommended! Better yet, simply don't use them.

Other tablets work by making you feel less hungry. It sounds great, but these tablets carry lots of side effects, including increased heart rate. This is something that is really *not* recommended if you are overweight, because your heart will already be under stress and you will very likely have high blood pressure. Do you *really* want to put your heart under even more strain?

If what I've written hasn't put you off using such medicines, I urge you to at least try embarking on a healthy weight loss regime for two months and see what happens before you rush off to ask your general practitioner for a prescription. I can guarantee you that if you commit 100 per cent to a new healthy eating and living regime, you will find that after two months, the desire to have such pills will be virtually non-existent. Just think carefully about what you are putting into your body.

Organisations & Websites

Whilst I would encourage you to carry out your own research and to seek the advice from a suitably qualified professional, bear in mind that the person whom you are seeking advice from should be *appropriately* qualified. If you do not know what a person's qualifications mean, ask them. If you are still unclear, ask your doctor or nurse. This is your health—you cannot afford to receive poor advice. You deserve the best.

Here is a list of some organisations and websites that may guide you in your quest to find further sources of help.

- *Power-Full Weight Loss*—This website offers further support and information for those embarking on a weight loss journey. http://www.powerfullweightloss.com info@powerfullweightloss.com
- *British Heart Foundation*—This is a charity organisation which offers advice as to how you can keep your heart healthy. It is also involved in the care of patients who have heart disease and in research in this field. internet@bhf.org.uk tel: 020 7554 0000
- *The British Dietetic Society*—This is a professional organisation for dieticians. The society website defines the role of the dietician, has essential food

fact information, and offers other essential advice. Info@bda.uk.com tel: 0121 200 8080

- *Weight Watchers*—This is a reputable weight loss organisation which has established itself across the world. It advises its members to follow a sensible, healthy eating plan that will allow them to lose unwanted weight at a sensible rate. Members attend weekly classes or follow an online programme. http://www.weightwatchers.co.uk/ uk.help@weightwatchers.co.uk

- *Scottish Slimmers*—This organisation is similar to Weight Watchers, in that it encourages healthy eating for weight loss. It is a smaller organisation but is well established and respected in Scotland. http://www.scottishslimmers.com/ (Freephone in UK): 0800 362636

- *Eating Disorders Association*—The Eating Disorders Association (known as BEAT), is a charity organisation that offers advice and support for sufferers and their families. help@b-eat.co.uk tel: 0845 634 1414

- *Overeaters Anonymous*—This is an organisation that offers support to compulsive overeaters by following a twelve-step programme. It is internationally recognised, with meetings being held in many countries. There is no joining fee, and anonymity of individuals who follow the programme is respected. http://www.oa.org

- *World Health Organisation (WHO)*—The WHO is a UN organisation which influences global health. Its website contains information about many different health issues, including nutrition and obesity. The information provided is both accurate and easy to read. http://www.who.int/en/

- *Life Coach*—A life coach can help you to focus on what you really want and find a way to make your goals a reality. A list of some life coaches can be found at http://www.findalifecoach.co.uk/index.htm

PART IV

So Who Am I?

Again I return to this question because I want to tell you who I am—or rather, I want to tell you all the important and significant stuff that a person wants to and sometimes needs to find out when she meets another person for the first time.

I was born Margaret Grace in Ayrshire, Scotland, in 1977. For as long as I can remember, I have had a sweet tooth and was described as being 'a good wee eater' by many adults when I was little. As a child, I found that no matter how hard I tried, I just could not resist indulging in sugary snacks—particularly chocolate.

I can recall a specific incident that occurred at Easter; I believe I was eight at the time. I had started to have strong cravings for chocolate and resented the fact that, as a child, I could not go out and buy it. (My mum and dad were always careful not to let my sister and me overindulge in chocolate over the Easter season). My sister had an Easter egg that she was going to keep until she felt like eating it. I really liked the little chocolates that came with her egg and I could not stop thinking about them.

I had not received a similar type of Easter egg, so there was no way that I could satisfy my cravings by having a secret indulgence of my own. Needless to say, it wasn't long before the thought of eating my sister's chocolates popped into my head! At first I was able to ignore the little voice in my head that said, 'You know you want that chocolate—eat it, eat it, *eat it!*' I was able to reason, reminding myself that as a child, I had no means of replacing the egg, and to take something without seeking permission was stealing. I also would not be able to justify *why* I had to take the chocolate.

Unfortunately, despite my logical reasoning *not* to steal my sister's treat, my cravings and urges got the better of me, and I took the chocolate. I decided that it would be best to prise open the egg with great care, therefore hiding any evidence of my interference. Then, I thought, when my sister would eventually come to open her egg, I would act surprised and suggest it was the result of a manufacturing fault! And so my plan was hatched—not bad for a eight year old, I thought!

Unfortunately, the moment I took the chocolate and put it into my mouth, I knew I had done wrong. All of a sudden, the plan that I had hatched in my mind did not seem to sound as convincing, and I started to dread being reprimanded. The time that lapsed between this moment of weakness and my sister discovering what had happened felt like an eternity. I realised that the only alternative I had to following through with my plan was to admit my wrong doing and ask for forgiveness. At eight years of age I, however, did not have the courage to do this. And so when my sister unwrapped her egg and discovered what had happened, she went mad! Immediately she pointed the finger at me and I tried really hard to deny it and to stick to my plan. I could not figure out what had prompted her to even suspect that I had been responsible in the first place. Surely I had exercised extreme care and had placed the packaging and wrappers back in their original state? Obviously not! The accusations continued, my suggestions as to what happened were ignored, and eventually I gave a tearful confession along with an apology and a request for forgiveness. I hung my head in shame and felt very embarrassed and exposed.

Once the tears had dried up, I reflected on my actions and the cause of them. I can recall finding some comfort in the fact that time would heal the pain and the shame.

I continued to live this double life up until my teenage years. I say 'unconsciously' because although my inner being was aware that my secret was wrong, I did not have the maturity to admit to myself that there was cause for concern. My cravings for sweet foods (in particular chocolate) seemed to intensify over the years.

As I developed into a teenager, I noticed that all I wanted to do was eat, and I resented the fact that I could not have complete control over what I could eat during meal times. I wanted to eat chocolate for breakfast, lunch and dinner! I had accepted that abstinence from chocolate had become impossible, and I found myself eating it between meal times. I felt resentment towards my parents for forcing me to eat proper meals and therefore consume calories that I would not have chosen had I been an adult. I knew that my chocolate habit was causing me to consume an unhealthy amount of fat and calories—the last thing I wanted to do was to eat unwanted calories forced upon me! Thankfully I exercised regularly, so my weight was never a major concern during my teenage years.

Once I left school, I went on to study podiatry at university. My university career was not as dazzling and as brilliant as I'd hoped it would be and so the bad eating habits continued, even after graduating, because I did not find myself to be in a job that I really enjoyed. In 1999 I was offered a position as a podiatrist in Aberdeen. This marked the beginning of a very dark period in my life. My inexperience of life, my immaturity and my low self-esteem made it virtually impossible for me to deal with difficulties at work and other challenges that most adults faced. I ended up feeling despair and hopelessness in a city in the north of Scotland, miles from Ayrshire, which I considered home. I felt as if I had no one to talk to and at this point, my biggest fear came true—I became obese. I basically gave up and couldn't cope. I couldn't cry, I couldn't scream, I couldn't talk. Inside, my mind screamed, 'Let me out, let me out!' But no one heard this, and so I felt trapped. The only thing I could do was eat . . . and eat . . . and eat. I put on 25kg in only four months.

I hated myself, my job, my boss, the city I was living in and what I had done and was doing to my family. I hated life and I wanted to kill myself, but I didn't have the guts to do it. I couldn't go into work and was signed off with 'stress and depression'. I felt really embarrassed at my actions. Even though I spoke to a counsellor and was put on anti-depressants, I still managed to put on another 20kg. At 157cm, my heaviest weight was a staggering 105kg!

Reflection

Desperate to change my situation, I decided to change my career and move to a new town. I decided on Dundee, where I had been accepted into a post-graduate nursing course. I had considered studying to become a teacher, but I had heard that competition to get onto the post graduate primary course was stiff, so I didn't even bother applying, thinking dejectedly to myself, 'I'll never get in'.

Quite clearly, lessons had not been learnt because it very quickly became apparent that the nursing career had been chosen simply as a means of getting me out of my previous situation. As a qualified podiatrist, I found it very difficult to adjust to the ways of nursing. Fear of letting my family down again, however, caused me to plod on in the hope that it would get better. As I slowly started to recover from the mental trauma experienced in Aberdeen, I realised that we all make mistakes in life and that as an adult, I had to accept responsibility for my mistakes. My subsequent actions required a lot of courage, considering that I had completed sixteen months of a twenty-four-month post-graduate course, but I took a deep breath, considered what my parents' worst reaction would be and then picked up the phone and told them I was quitting the course.

Naturally my parents were not happy. I felt that I had let them down (again), but I stood firm in my decision knowing that I had not let myself down. I had at last started to listen to my instincts and consider what *my* needs were. I was starting to grow up and slowly recover.

Sadly this recovery was hindered by the fact that I had still not managed to lose weight—I was still a hefty size twenty-four, and because I was determined that I was *not* going to go back to podiatry, I found myself to be unemployed. Money was a real issue, and it took a lot of effort to lift myself out of the dark cloud that hovered over me. It was a battle that lasted eight months.

Eventually an old colleague, who had a private clinic, was able to offer me some days as a podiatrist in her practice. This offer was a saving grace and although she could only offer me three and a half days each week and I had to travel 60km to and from work (by train, because I had not passed my driving test), I was *just* able to make ends meet and was finally starting to see some evidence of real hope. I knew that the old Mags was in me somewhere and I was determined to reveal her again. I remember thinking at that time how bizarre it was that some of my friends had never known me to be at a normal weight.

As many things in my life started to improve, I knew that there was still the huge issue of my weight, which had to be addressed. As a health professional, I recognised the signs and symptoms of pre-diabetes and I knew that my health was suffering. I found myself getting breathless, my hair was very dull and dry and my skin was spotty and greasy. I was snoring, I was struggling to bend down and I had bad breath. I could hardly fit in a seat in a plane or train, I struggled to wipe my bottom after going to the toilet and I struggled to step over the side of the bath to get into the shower. I also experienced excessive sweating, headaches, painful periods and I had bouts of diarrhoea and extreme tiredness! The list could go on and on, but the symptoms that really spurred me on to change were the fact that I had high blood pressure and constantly had to go to the toilet during the night. My urine had a strong odour and was a dark yellow, colour which also concerned me. These symptoms suggested the early onset of type II diabetes and I knew only too well that this could lead to both limb and sight loss and other problems. The third symptom related to my mental health was that I had zero confidence and self-esteem. At only twenty-four years old, I was a morbidly obese catastrophe. I *had* to change.

December 2004 marked a period of reflection and a real commitment to take action. I realised that I could not continue to exist as I was and if I were to change, I would have to commit to it with 100 per cent effort. I would not deceive myself but would be realistic and proactive. Coincidently, at this time I received a free magazine through the post from

Scottish Slimmers. I flipped through the pages looking at before-and-after pictures of successful slimmers, wishing that the pictures were of me and that the whole weight-loss process was 'that easy'.

I came across a success story that caught my interest. It was about a woman who was from the north east of Scotland and worked in a chip shop. She had lost a staggering amount of weight (between 40-50kg, as far as I can remember). I found myself admiring this woman's strength and determination because I knew that a chippie (the commonly known name for a chip shop in the west coast of Scotland) would not be an easy environment to work in whilst trying to adopt a healthier diet. For those of you who are unaware, the local chippie in Scotland not only serves fish and chips, but it also serves fried sausages, chicken, pizza, black pudding, haggis, pies, chocolate, crisps, sweets, and tins of juice! Yes, the local chippie really is a heart attack haven!

Besides admiring this woman for successfully rising to her challenge, I noticed a little voice in my head that was saying, 'Well, if she could do that, you can too!' The voice just seemed to get louder and made more comments like, 'It will be easier for you because you don't work in a chip shop. You're just the same as that woman. Your body's no different, so what's stopping you? What have you got to lose aside from weight? You might as well give it a go. You never know—it might work, and you could be thinner!' The voice didn't go away—it just got louder and I felt that I had no other choice but to act accordingly.

My study of physiology and medicine as part of my degree, combined with my personal interest in nutrition, exercise and diet, allowed me to foster a sensible approach that was healthy and easy to stick to. I also understood what a safe rate of weight loss would be. Considering this knowledge and the fact that I wanted to keep my new regime a secret for various reasons, and that money was tight, I decided to embark upon this journey alone and did not join any slimming clubs.

I decided to give myself one month to see what would happen. If, at the end of January, I had committed myself 100 per cent to a change in lifestyle and had lost a significant amount of weight (3kg, possibly more), I would review the situation and decide what further actions I could possibly take in February. If, however, after committing myself 100 per cent to a new regime, I had not lost anything, I would most likely shelve my plans.

I resolved not to put myself under any pressure. No foods were banned and I decided not to force myself to do any exercise. I think that it was for this reason that I can remember feeling quietly confident and determined that things *would* change for the better. As a health professional, I understood that my morbidly obese state meant that it would be sensible for me to start off with a higher daily calorie allowance than someone who was just 'overweight' and my weight loss would be more rapid and noticeable on the scales to start with because the more obese you are, the more fluid you lose when first embarking on a healthier diet programme.

I quietly and confidently expected myself to lose 3kg easily in January, then another 2-3kg a month later. As it was, I found myself constantly urinating in January, losing a staggering 6kg in the first month! Needless to say, this motivated me to continue my regime, include exercise into it and I dropped from 105kg to 60kg in twelve months!

My determination, resolve to remain focussed and realistic expectations allowed me to not only reduce my body fat percentage from 46 per cent to 24 per cent, my BMI from 44 to 22 and my weight from 105 to 60kg; but I also became more confident and achieved other goals that were related to my weight. For example, I completed a marathon in Belfast. This was a huge achievement on my part because I had previously *hated* running!

It was during this special year that I also passed my driving test after four previous failed attempts and I secured a place on a post-graduate teaching course. During my period of unemployment and then working at my friend's private practice, I carefully considered in which direction my career should turn. Even if I had wanted to return to podiatry full time, which I knew I didn't (although I was starting to realise that I enjoyed using my medical knowledge and some other skills associated with podiatry), I could not do so because I had started to develop quite serious bouts of repetitive strain injury in my right wrist. Initially I applied for the teaching course the year before I embarked on my exciting weight loss journey and I had failed to secure a place. However, as I started to lose weight and after I passed my driving test, I found that I was determined to try again for the following academic year. This time I was successful and qualified as a teacher ten months later!

There were very few teaching jobs in Scotland, so I decided to opt for a job in a school in Saudi Arabia. I had a wonderful experience and stayed in the capital city of Riyadh for three years. I then worked in Abu Dhabi for a year before moving to Dubai, where I now work as a medical instructor. My life in Dubai is amazing! I am very busy and have met many interesting and inspirational people. I play squash regularly, work out at the gym and play my flute in a music group.

My slimming success was celebrated and shared with not only close friends and family, but I even had the privilege of being featured in a national glossy magazine and was awarded a substantial sum in shopping vouchers!

You Reached Your Target . . .
What Next?

Congratulations! Now that you've reached your target, how can you ensure that you maintain a healthy weight and size?

If you refer back to the section 'What's Right for Me', you will be able to determine how many calories you can eat on a daily basis by working out the simple calculation described. Just remember that although you are now able to increase your daily calorie consumption, you must still eat a healthy diet and continue to exercise regularly. Continue also to read inspirational and exercise related magazines and books and socialise with like-minded people.

I would like to wish you all the very best. Here's to a healthy and happy future!

Bibliography

- Baic, S.; Rinzler, C. A. (2006). *Nutrition for Dummies.* England: John Wiley & Sons, Ltd.
- Peters, M. (ed.); Davidson, S.; Preston, P.; Williams, F. (medical advisors) (2002). *The British Medical Association Illustrated Medical Dictionary.* London: Dorling Kindersley Ltd.
- Collins UK. (2003). *Collins Gem Calorie Counter* Glasgow: Harper Collins Publishers.
- Delaney, L. (2008). *Secrets of a Former Fat Girl.* New York: Plume Penguin Group.
- Edgson, V.; Marber, I. (1999). *The Food Doctor— Healing Foods for Minds and Body.* London: Collins & Brown Ltd.
- *Weight Watchers Magazine.* (August 2009, issue 636). River Publishing Ltd.

Internet Sites

- Wikipedia—The Free Encyclopedia. (accessed 30 September 2009) *Body Fat Percentage—Wikipedia.* http://en.wikipedia.org/wiki/Body_fat_percentage.
- BBC. (accessed 29 September 2009) *News Health.* http://news.bbc.co.uk/2/hi/health
- National Health Service, U.K. (accessed 20 October 2009) *Lose Weight* http://www.nhs.uk/Livewell/loseweight
- British Heart Foundation. (accessed 29 September 2009) *Heart Health* http://www.bhf.org.uk
- Tesco Diets. (accessed 30 September 2009) *Lose Weight, Love Life* http://www.tescodiets.com.
- Healthy Check Systems. (accessed 18 October 2009) *Body Fat* http://www.healthchecksystems.com/bodyfat.htm.
- Answers.com. (accessed 27 July 2009) *Food Pyramid* http://www.answers.com/topic/food-guide-pyramid

Appendix 1

Weight Loss Progress Table

Date	Weight

Date	Weight

Weight Loss Progress Graph

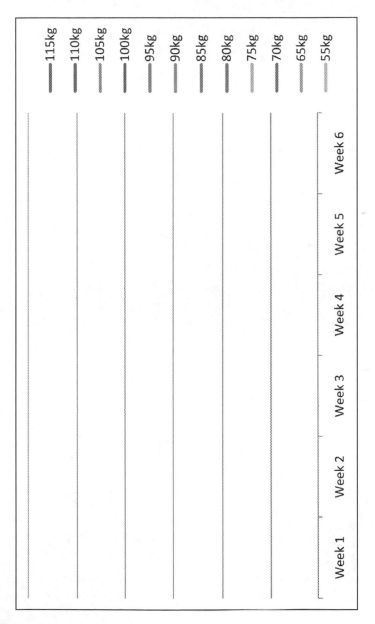

115kg 110kg 105kg 100kg 95kg 90kg 85kg 80kg 75kg 70kg 65kg 55kg

Week 1 Week 2 Week 3 Week 4 Week 5 Week 6

Change the weeks to specific dates as required.

Appendix 2

Measurement & Waist-Hip Ratio Table

Date	Left Thigh	Right Thigh	Hips	Waist	Chest	Right Upper Arm	Left Upper Arm	Waist-Hip Ratio

Date	Left Thigh	Right Thigh	Hips	Waist	Chest	Right Upper Arm	Left Upper Arm	Waist-Hip Ratio